27(Twenty Seven)

Great Health

Benefits Of Clean

Water

Olatundun Solomon

olatundunsolomon

@gmail.com

1. Prevent Cholera :

The microorganism

that cause cholera

is prevented by

drinking clean water.

2. Prevent Diarrhea:

The microorganism

that cause diarrhea

is prevented by

drinking clean water.

3. Prevent

Dysentery: The

microorganism that

cause dysentery is

prevented by

drinking clean water.

4. Prevent skin

infection: The

microorganism that

can cause skin

infection through

dirty water can be

prevented by

drinking clean water

and bathing with

clean water.

5. Can assist to

prevent wrinkles:

Drinking enough

clean water can

hydrate the skin

and there by

preventing wrinkles.

Especially in

children and young

adults.

6. Cause hydration:
When there is
dehydration of the
body, drinking clean
water can cause

hydration of the

body.

7. Can treat

constipation: When

the faeces is too

hard and it can not

come out of the

body. Drinking

water can soften it.

It can assist it to

come out.

8. Can help in

preventing arthritis:

Drinking water can

assist in the

lubrication of the

joints. It can assist

in preventing

arthritis.

9. Can help in
detoxifying the
body.

10. Can help in the
removal of
microorganisms

from clothes by

washing the clothes

with soap and

water.

11. Can help to prevent kidney stones. Drinking enough water can help kidney stones not to accumulate in the kidneys.

12. Can assist the

heart to function

normally.

13. Can assist for

the tongue to

produce enough

saliva. It assist in

making the tongue

wet.

14. Can assist the

brain function

normally.

15. Can prevent headache, by lowering high temperature of the body. For example, drinking cold water

when the

temperature of the

environment is high.

16. Can assist in

making the high

body temperature

to become normal.

By drinking cold

water.

17. Water can assist

the body

electrolytes to be

balance.

18. Water can make

the skin appearance

to be fine by

lubricating it.

19. Water can help

in digestion of food

in the body.

20. Water can help

to assist in replacing

water loss after

sweating.

21. Water can assist

to make the hair

look fine because of

lubrication of the

body.

22. Water can assist

to prevent friction

in the eyes by

lubricating the eyes.

23. Water can assist

the blood to

function well. This

makes the blood to

not be too thick.

24. Water can assist

in urination.

25. Drink warm

water during cold

weather. It can

make the body

warm during cold
weather.

26. It is good for
pregnant woman to
drink enough water.
The pregnant

woman and the

fetus inside her

needs water.

27. Swimming in

clean water can be

as a form of

exercise that can

keep the body fit.